Re-Medispa

by Renata Ciszek APN-BC

Re-Medispa
Copyright © 2017 by Renata Ciszek APN-BC

I am an Adult Nurse Practitioner with more than 15 years of experience in the healthcare system. I am writing this book to break a taboo about health problems that women are too embarrassed to talk about. These problems are the results of natural physiological changes that women go through as they age.

I strongly believe in treating these issues with feminine rejuvenation treatments. These are treatments for women with many forms of sexual dysfunction.

The main issues I see women suffering with are stress incontinence and sexual dysfunction. Stress incontinence is a condition where women leak urine when they exercise, sneeze, lift weights or laugh. It's caused by a weakening of the pelvic floor muscle, or bladder muscle. The common treatments available are just not that effective. And the medications for these conditions have so many side effects that women do not take them.

Another problem that is almost a taboo topic, is sexual dysfunction. Sexual dysfunction can present in many ways. It can be that a woman is not able to achieve orgasm during sexual intercourse, or has decreased libido. Another situation can be vaginal dryness that prevents women from enjoying sexual contact, or causing pain during intercourse.

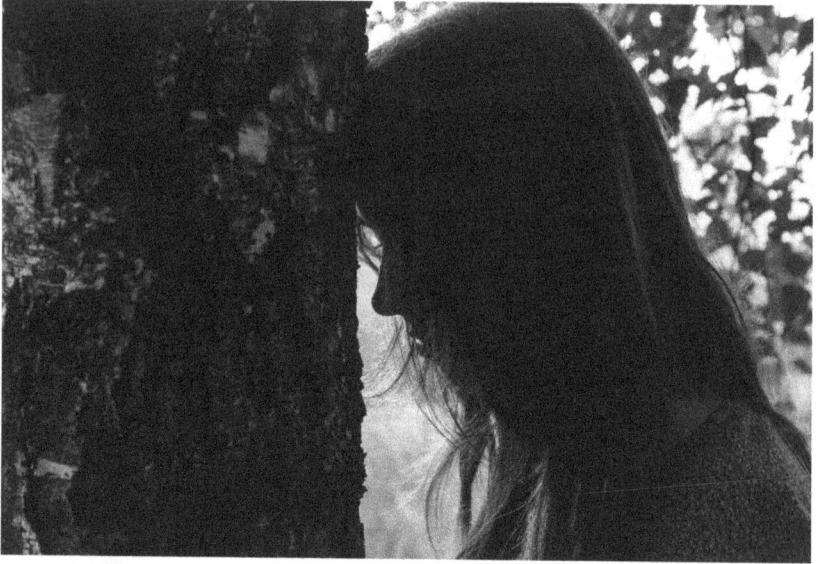

I personally know women – I am thinking of one in particular – who actually divorced her husband because she had so much pain during sexual intercourse. She didn't feel she could talk to him about it, and no health care providers were able to help her. Because she was avoiding sexual contact, he felt they were no longer attracted to each other, and that caused conflict between them, which led to divorce.

After undergoing feminine rejuvenation treatments, women who previously could not climax, start having intense orgasms for the first time. Women who leaked urine when laughing, sneezing, coughing or exercising find their problem resolved. Women who had vaginal dryness experience the opposite. These are life-changing treatments for women, which makes them a necessity and not just an option.

The treatments allow women to feel in control again, and sexy. When you feel good, it shows in your body language, voice and facial expressions. The whole world looks better and personal problems seem less significant. I have had clients come in to my med spa crying and hoping I can help them. One client's husband told her that she was "too loose" and did not satisfy him anymore. Sex had always been important in their marriage and it was devastating to her. She was treated with laser and O-Shot, and when she called me a month later, crying again, this time they were tears of happiness. She felt that the treatments saved her marriage. Imagine how many husbands don't tell their wives how they feel about their sex life but, instead, cheat with a different lover.

How did you get started doing these treatments?

It started with my own sexual dysfunction. I was a frustrated woman suffering from sexual dysfunction. It was really hard for me to achieve orgasm. I kept searching for answers but kept finding conflicting information. One source said it was my fault and I need to be more relaxed, to "let it go" in bed, etc. I tried that, but it didn't work. Other sources blamed the partner for not knowing a woman's anatomy well enough, and not asking questions.

Then I came across research saying that 40% of women have some form of sexual dysfunction, which made me realize I was not alone. I knew there had to be a treatment for my problem and I just needed to find it.

However, I could not understand why (since one out of every three women had sexual dysfunction) no one talked about it. Why was it a taboo topic?

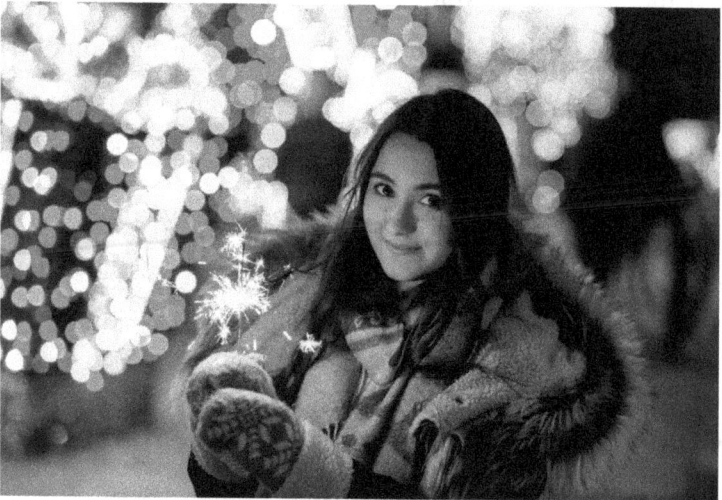

I've been in the medical field for over 15 years but I could not recall one time that I spoke with my female patients about sexual dysfunction. I didn't know women suffered from this issue. It was almost expected that when you were older, you leaked urine. I realized there are so many women with sexual dysfunction, or stress incontinence, who just don't talk about it. They're either too embarrassed to talk about it or they have nobody to talk to. So, I decided I needed to break this taboo and help women, especially since there is help available for these problems.

I really started talking about it after I attended a chamber of commerce meeting and, as a medical professional, presented about sexual dysfunction and available treatments. I was told not to come back, and that I didn't "match the group." The group was mostly men who did not want to know that their wives might suffer from some form of dysfunction. These men wanted to pretend their wives don't have any problems.

I wondered: if these 100 men have perfect wives, why do 60% of couples get divorced? Statistically, couples with a great sex life report better life satisfaction and they stay together longer. Maybe those "happy wives" got tired of pretending they have an orgasm every time they have sex. Or maybe husbands did not have the courage to communicate that their sex life was not the same, and found someone to meet their needs on the side.

I feel strongly that women need to know they are not alone and that there is treatment available. One of the reasons some topics are taboo, I believe, is a lack of education about the subject. I am hoping to break the silence.

In my research, I learned about Dr. Runels, who invented the O-Shot procedure. I read his patients' reviews and it sounded as though the procedure truly works. I contacted Dr. Runels and went to Alabama for training with him.

Then I learned about Femilift lasers, too. I read that some physicians combine the laser treatment with the O-Shot procedure to obtain optimal results. I called one of the companies and insisted on trying the treatment on one of my clients that suffered from vaginal dryness. A week later, my client called and said she no longer had friction between her legs when she walked. She felt the treatment was working. I purchased the vaginal rejuvenation laser and started offering both treatments together.

Why do women suffer from sexual dysfunction? Is it a part of aging?

There are many forms of sexual dysfunction. Some women suffer from stress incontinence, some from lack of orgasm and others have either painful intercourse or vaginal dryness. I see all forms of dysfunction; however, the most common complaint I hear from my clients is stress incontinence.

Stress incontinence occurs when the muscle and tissue that supports the bladder, which regulates the release of urine, weakens. In a healthy individual, the bladder expands as it fills with urine. There is a muscle around the opening of the bladder, a sphincter, that stays squeezed closed to prevent urine from leaking. When that muscle weakens, anything that puts pressure on the abdominal or pelvic muscles – like bending over, sneezing or laughing – can put pressure on the bladder and cause urine to leak.

Childbirth is the most common cause of the pelvic and sphincter muscle weakening. A baby passing through the vaginal canal can cause tissue or nerve damage. That damage can be apparent soon after delivery, or it can show up many years later. The O-Shot rejuvenates the tissue and nerves damaged during delivery and makes the muscles stronger.

Another cause of stress incontinence is hormonal changes, especially estrogen. Normally, estrogen helps our pelvic floor to be strong and stretchy, which gives us greater control over our bladder. As we age, though, our estrogen level decreases, which causes vaginal tissue to lose its thickness, elasticity and natural lubrication. It also makes our pelvic muscles weaker, contributing to stress incontinence. This is why addressing the hormone level is as important as administering the O-Shot injection or Femilift treatment.

Cancer treatments such as chemotherapy can also lead to low estrogen and a decrease in vaginal lubrication. My female client with the severe vaginal dryness (to the point of having pain when she walked due to friction) did not want to take the amount of estrogen recommended by her gynecologist because estrogen can be carcinogenic as well as leading to weight gain and bloating. It's why many women don't want to take replacement estrogen.

A week after her first treatment, she called and told me she could walk without friction and pain. After her second treatment, she felt even better and reported that sex was no longer painful and she didn't need to use lubricants anymore. After receiving the third treatment, all her symptoms were resolved.

Something else that can contribute to stress incontinence is high-impact exercise over time, as it puts pressure on the pelvic muscles. One of my med spa clients exercised heavily with a personal trainer, and one day she noticed her pants were wet while doing squat exercises. She had the O-Shot injection and after one month, she reported to me that she no longer leaked urine.

Another common complaint I hear from women is a lack of orgasm from sexual intercourse. There can be many causes for that condition and a global approach is needed. In many cases, there is decreased blood flow to the vagina and clitoris, which can delay or stop orgasm entirely. This is why the O-Shot and Femilift laser treatments are so effective, as both treatments rejuvenate the vaginal tissue and that means more blood flow, more sensitivity and stronger orgasms.

Hormones need to be checked as well, since an imbalance can affect orgasm. Hormones are chemical messengers that cause the reaction of every tissue in our body. The hormones that can affect a woman's sexual pleasure include testosterone, thyroid, estrogen, prolactin, progesterone and oxytocin. For a woman, testosterone and thyroid function play a major role in their sex drive. Women who take birth control pills see their testosterone levels drop as a side effect of the pill, and the drop in testosterone can lead to weight gain, migraines and decreased sexual function.

Estrogen plays a primary role in vaginal mucosa health. That's why when estrogen decreases, women complain about dryness and laxity. Unfortunately, estrogen can be carcinogenic and it leads to weight gain and bloating. Therefore, many women do not want to take replacement estrogen.

A prolactin level that's too high can cause decreased libido, lack of arousal and difficulty with orgasm. Progesterone affects libido more than estrogen but less than testosterone.

Oxytocin is released during orgasm. Some women make less oxytocin than others. Research showed that women who have difficulty achieving orgasm have lower levels of oxytocin.

Hormones are a huge part of orgasm, and hormonal imbalance can cause women to struggle with it and with their sex drive. Statistically, 40% of women suffer from lack of orgasm. Therefore, a practitioner needs to address both the hormonal role and vaginal health of his or her female patient.

What treatments are available for these women, and how do you do them?

We use two feminine rejuvenation treatments in the med spa – the O-Shot and feminine laser rejuvenation. We can use them alone or we can combine them for optimal results. After we present the benefits of each, a lot of women choose both treatments.

With O-Shot, we inject Platelet Rich Plasma (PRP) into the roof of the vagina and clitoris. Here's how it is done: first, the medical professional draws blood from the client. Then they place the blood in an FDA-approved centrifuge. The centrifuge we use in the med spa is the EmCyte centrifuge. The blood is spun twice, at different speeds. The end result is that the red blood cells go to the

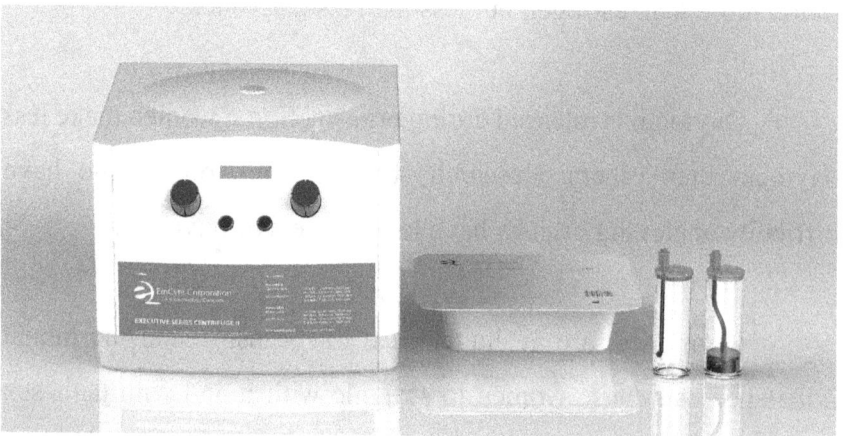

bottom and platelets are left at the top. The practitioner then activates the platelets with calcium chloride and injects the PRP into the specific area in the vagina and clitoris.

The activated PRP releases growth factors that stimulate and recruit stem cells to grow new, healthier tissue that is more oxygenated and better innervated. This also produces new collagen and elastin production. Elastin is responsible for allowing tissues in the body to "snap back" to their original shape after being stretched, and collagen gives skin and tissue their strength. For women who suffer from stress incontinence caused by pelvic muscle weakness, the new collagen and elastin is what makes her able to hold urine.

The treatment was invented by Dr. Charles Runels. I was privileged to be personally trained by Dr. Runels in Alabama. We have already done over 100 O-Shots in the clinic and our success rate is very high.

Another treatment that we use is the Femilift laser. It's a CO_2 laser that works by creating micro channels, about .5 mm deep, inside the vaginal wall. This stimulates collagen production and elastin. After three treatments, the vagina is tighter and there is more sexual pleasure, tissue tone is restored and the blood flow is better. This, in turn, increases lubrication and strengthens the supporting ligaments surrounding the bladder and urethra. This means women are able to hold urine as they used to, and sexual pleasure during intercourse is enhanced as well. By combining the O-Shot with the Femilift treatment, women get the best results possible.

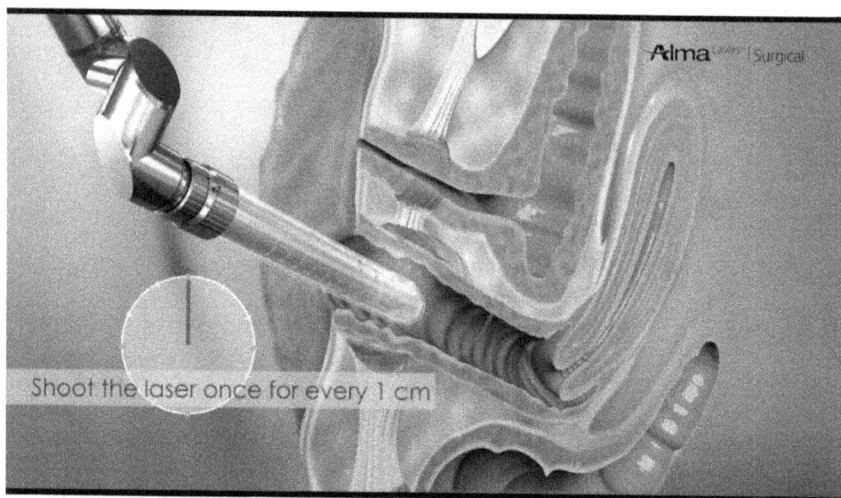

Shoot the laser once for every 1 cm

How do you determine which treatment is better for any particular woman?

Consultation is key. If a woman's main concern is lack of orgasm, then the O-Shot is great for that and we inject the PRP into the clitoris. The Femilift laser works only inside the vagina and does not treat the clitoris. O-Shot is great for stress incontinence as well – however, I've found that if we combine the O-Shot with the Femilift laser, results last longer and a woman notices the results quicker. After all, she is getting a "double whammy." I also recommend both treatments for a woman who is not able to hold urine and constantly needs to wear pads. Both treatments work great for vaginal dryness and laxity, so for those conditions the female patient can choose which treatment she prefers. Undergoing both treatments gives more optimal results.

Does it hurt? Do you feel pain, and can you resume normal activities right after the treatment?

Both treatments are very well tolerated. Even though we use a needle to inject PRP into the vagina for the O-Shot, the injection does not hurt because we use numbing cream for 20 minutes prior. For the clitoris, we use numbing cream as well, and right before the injection we use an ice cube to numb the area even more. We can also inject Lidocaine into the hood of the clitoris if a woman is really afraid of pain. However, a lot of times this is not necessary.

When we use the Femilift laser for vaginal rejuvenation, it doesn't hurt at all. I can speak for Femilift as that is the one I have been using. The treatment is so well-tolerated that some women are surprised when I tell them we are done with the treatment.

I was actually surprised that the CO_2 laser does not hurt in the vagina, since it is very painful when used to treat the face. Looking more deeply into this, I learned that the vagina sheath has very few nerve endings, which is why it does not hurt during the treatment. The most sensitive part of the vagina, which has the most touch-sensitive nerve endings, is about 1 cm farther from the entrance. That is also the area where we inject the O-Shot, but we do not go there with the laser.

There is really no downtime. You can have sexual intercourse right away after the O-Shot, and some women actually report extreme arousal after the treatment. The hyper-sexual response is a result of growth factors being released from the platelets and causing enhanced blood flow and better sensitivity. That response may last for a couple of days until the body completely absorbs the injected PRP. That's when the regeneration process begins. Women notice more permanent benefits about three weeks after the shot, and it takes about three months to get the maximum effect.

Woman can resume normal daily activity after the vaginal laser treatment; however, we recommend no sexual intercourse for at least three days post-treatment. Some women might have minimal spotting for a day or two, but there are no other issues. Before the treatment, we recommend women have a gynecological exam, including pap smear, to make sure there are no medical problems contributing to the issues she came in to fix. Also, we require a pregnancy test the day of the procedure. The patient can do it at home or we can do it in the office.

How long do the effects of these treatments last, and when do you need to repeat them?

After the O-Shot injection, it takes about four to five weeks for the rejuvenation process to take place. Then the O-Shot can be repeated. It takes about three months for maximum effect. The treatment can last a year or two; it depends on the individual. There are cases where a woman has one injection of O-Shot and two years later she is still satisfied with her results. The results vary depending on the person and they are not guaranteed. However, overall about 90% of women nationwide achieve satisfaction from the results.

In our practice, I am proud to say that 95% of our clients are happy with the results. So far, I only had one woman that did not respond to the O-Shot and I am currently treating her with the Femilift laser. She has two more treatments to go, so I do not know her outcome yet. This woman had a hysterectomy; she is in her 50s and her main problem is lack of orgasm. She is also seeing a doctor for hormone replacement therapy and just recently adjusted the dose.

The Femilift laser treatment is recommended every month for three months total, and then one maintenance treatment every year thereafter. The effect can last several years.

Most patients feel tighter and have a more lubricated vagina wall after the first treatment. It takes weeks to rebuild collagen and elastin, so treatments are spaced one month apart to allow for that time of rejuvenation. Patients are instructed to perform Kegel exercises at home to further expedite and enhance the ongoing tissue remodeling and collagen contraction occurring after the treatment. Hormonal levels need to be monitored by the provider, as well, for optimal results.

The final outcome is more lubrication, enhanced sexual sensation for both women and men, resolution of urine leakage and no more pain during intercourse. Women feel sexier, more confident and happier, and men benefit from that as well, if you know what I mean. Just like the saying, "Happy wife, happy life."

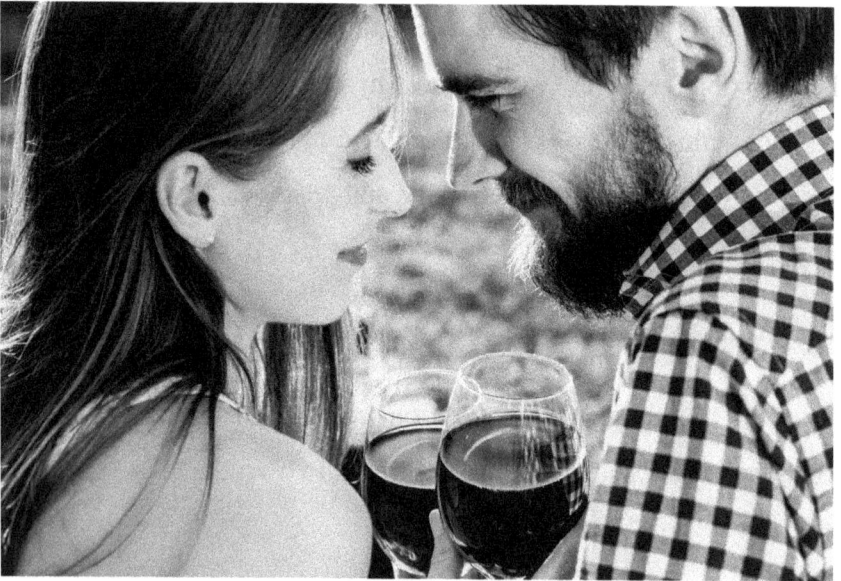

Are there situations or conditions under which these treatments are not recommended?

Yes. Women are required to have a complete OB/GYN exam, including pap smear, within a month of the treatment and a pregnancy test within 24 hrs. If the pap smear is abnormal or if there is any active HPV/herpes, the treatment is not performed. Also, if there is any undiagnosed vaginal bleeding, or if the woman has her menstrual cycle, we do not perform the treatment. Unexplained vaginal bleeding could be a serious condition; therefore, we don't want to mask anything with the laser.

Pregnancy is another condition during which we would not perform the treatment. Chronic corticosteroid therapy and uncontrolled diabetes slow down the healing process; therefore, treatment with laser is not recommended for people with those conditions. Gynecological cancer is another condition that would prevent us from performing this treatment. Depending on the severity, clients with collagen disease or any disease affecting the immune system may not be able to have the laser treatment done.

The O-Shot, on the other hand, is a very safe procedure and there are only a few situations that would prevent us from performing it. The main one is a patient having a low platelets level, since we need platelets to be concentrated five to six times more than normal after the spin. Also, there is a higher risk of bleeding when your platelets are low. There is also a minimal risk of urinary tract infection. The needle is very small, almost the size of diabetic insulin needles, so there is no problem with healing.

What is the success rate?

In 2015, there was a study done in Europe where 86% reported improvement in orgasmic response, 75% noticed improvement in vaginal lubrication and painful intercourse, and overall, 93.4% of patients described the procedure as "excellent" or "good."

In many cases, I combine the O-Shot with the Femilift laser treatment in order to get maximum effect, and the success rate of both procedures is about 90%. There is no procedure that works 100%, of course, but I do think our satisfaction rate is high. In one case, I had to send a client to someone specializing in Chinese medicine as I felt she had a problem with an emotional block that wasn't allowing her to achieve orgasm. She was able to get the help she needed and she enjoyed her sex life like never before.

How much do the procedures cost?

Treatment prices differ depending on the location of the med spa. The inventor of the O-Shot procedure priced the treatment at $1,200, and we are not allowed to discount. Practitioners can charge a higher price, but not less than $1,200. I have seen the cost as high as $3,000, especially in California where the cost of living is higher.

The price for the Femilift laser treatment varies as well. The company recommends the price to be between $2,400 and $3,000 for three treatments one month apart. The actual price depends on the place offering the treatment. When I combine the two treatments, I give a higher discount on the Femilift treatment so it is more affordable for clients. It's all about helping women, and we work within their budget so they can afford it.

Are these treatments FDA-approved? Are they safe in the long run?

This is the most common question my clients ask. The Femilift laser was approved by the FDA about three years ago. The first laser that came to the U.S. was called Mona Lisa. It came from Europe where results were so impressive it got attention worldwide.

The Femilift company claims that its Femilift laser is the gold standard, as it is more precise and provides more comfortable treatments than any other lasers on the market. The settings and number of treatments were designed based on studies and they were proven to be very effective and safe.

The O-Shot procedure does not require FDA approval since there is no drug involved. The client's own blood is used for the treatment; therefore, it is a very safe procedure.

However, the centrifuge machine used to spin the blood needs to be FDA-approved. We are using the EmCyte centrifuge machine in our med spa. It is considered one of the best on the market, giving a concentration of five to six times the platelets' normal content level. A higher platelets concentration means more growth factors are released and there is more stem cell activation.

You can compare the procedure to a surgeon sewing a wound. The sutures he uses need to be FDA-approved, but the FDA does not tell the surgeon how to close the wound. He learned that in medical school.

The providers of O-Shot are all trained by the inventor, who is a medical doctor. It is a specific method of injecting PRP into the vagina and is protected by U.S. patent and trademark law. All providers are listed on the O-Shot website. The trademark identifies providers (medical doctors, nurse practitioners and physician assistants) that meet the required standards and may legally advertise with the name "O-Shot" or "Orgasm Shot." This does not promise women a perfect outcome but it does promise an excellent standard of care. People who say the O-Shot is not FDA-approved don't really understand the procedure and what is involved.

The only long-term effect of both treatments is a rejuvenated vagina, a better sex life and more life satisfaction. Why would anybody object to that, especially if it is a safe procedure? Don't forget that a tighter vagina also means more pleasure for men, so both sides benefit from the treatments.

Do all providers need to use the same equipment for O-Shot? Can providers use other centrifuges?

Yes, there is other equipment on the market that is FDA-approved. However, based on research in which platelets were compared using different machines, two stand out – Harvest and EmCyte. The difference between those two is price. With Harvest, you pay more for the machine but the kit costs less. For EmCyte, it is the opposite. The machine costs less but the kit for each use is more expensive. In the long run, it is more cost-efficient to have the Harvest centrifuge machine. The platelets concentration, after the second spin, is very consistent. Dr. Runels, inventor of the procedure, requires that the machine be FDA-approved and the concentration of Platelet Rich Plasma (PRP) be at least five times normal level.

How do I choose the provider? What questions should I ask?

To ensure the O-Shot is done by a certified provider, check the O-Shot provider list. Every person on that list was personally trained by the inventor, Dr. Runels. It also means that provider is using FDA-approved equipment and is following standard procedure.

I often get the question, "How long have you been doing the procedure?" When I say about two years, people respond, "Oh, so you're not that experienced." I remind women that it's a new procedure, so all providers have been doing the treatment about the same amount of time. I also encourage potential clients to look at online reviews and our clients' testimonials. The clients' satisfaction is our top priority.

Do you recommend women undergo either of these treatments as preventative treatment, or should they wait until problems start?

Women have the tendency to not really take care of themselves until there is a problem. What I see a lot in women is guilt. "Oh, why would I spend money on this treatment when I have to provide for my children? I have to pay for college!" So no, women do not come for preventative treatments, which is interesting to me because they do spend money on Botox and fillers.

On the other hand, many women don't know that treatments like O-Shot and Femilift are available to them. One of my patients was lifting weights when her personal trainer pointed out that the patient's pants were wet. The patient, who did not even feel it, was so embarrassed and left the gym. She called me in a panic, not knowing what just happened. She had her first occurrence of stress incontinence. I discussed treatment options with her: the O-Shot vs. Femilift vs. both. She decided to have the O-Shot. She has not had stress incontinence since undergoing the treatment.

I feel women should have more education about this topic. If I were not in the medical field, my client probably would have kept the incident to herself, thinking that it was "part of the aging process." It affects women's self-esteem, confidence and sexuality, and if you don't feel good about yourself, then you're not happy. If you're not happy, that affects how you interact with your husband and your children. So when we offer these treatments to a woman, it's not just to treat the problem. Indirectly we treat the entire family, because there is a saying that when the woman is happy, the family is happy. Happy wife, happy life.

I know a woman who divorced her husband because she felt he didn't satisfy her sexually. She was blaming it on him. It never occurred to her that she might be the problem. Then she had another partner and had the same issue. She went to her doctor, who educated her about the changes in the vagina after age 40, and available treatments.

That was my exact story, too. After changing a sexual partner and still not being sexually satisfied, I thought it was my partner not trying hard enough. Then I changed partners again, hoping for a better outcome, but this kept happening. Eventually, you get to the conclusion that maybe it is not "them." Maybe it's you. That was the reason I became involved in vaginal rejuvenation and orgasm in the first place.

Is there anything else women can do to improve their sexual health?

Number one is to be open with your partner if your needs are not being met. We only live once so let's enjoy life to the fullest. We women work so hard all day and we deserve to be rewarded at night.

In life, there has to be balance. "You give and you receive." If you just give all the time, your cup eventually becomes empty and that makes you frustrated and angry. You start playing the blame game and it can even break up a marriage.

On the other hand, if you have balance in your personal life you are better able to deal with everyday challenges and your overall life satisfaction is better.

When I was going to training on the O-Shot, there was a physician in our group that decided to go through O-Shot training to help his wife. When his wife first told him she could not achieve orgasm during intercourse, he told himself, "I can fix her; I'm a doctor." However, no matter how much he tried he was not successful.

Finally, he realized that it was not him; it was that his wife needed more than just regular sexual stimulation. Imagine if she had never told him she was not satisfied but instead kept pretending to enjoy sex. Eventually, she would have gotten tired of playing and started avoiding sexual contact with her husband. That may have led to arguments and maybe cheating, etc. Sometimes men cheat just to prove themselves and their ego.

I recommend always being open with your partner. Otherwise, you cannot be upset about anybody else but just yourself.

Are there other treatments along the same lines as O-Shot?

Yes. Platelet Rich Plasma (PRP), which is used for the O-Shot, can be used on other parts of the body. Since concentrated platelets release growth factors, which in turn activate stem cells, they can be used for any part of the body needing regeneration. They can be used for hair regrowth, facials and facelifts as well as breast lifts and P-Shots for men with erectile dysfunction. Our med spa specializes in these treatments as well, and I was also personally trained in these procedures by the inventor, Dr. Runels.

Any final advice for women out there? They're our sisters and our moms. Any other thoughts?

Any time they have any issues they know are not normal – and it doesn't matter if it's stress incontinence, sexual dysfunction or something else – they should talk to their medical provider.
But sometimes the providers are not aware of new technology like O-Shot or lasers. Some urologists still don't know what the O-Shot is.

If a woman is suffering enough to see a provider about her problem, and he says there is nothing that can be done, she should not stop there. Do your research and see what is available.

Technology has advanced so much and there is no reason that women must suffer.

If people are interested in learning more, how can they reach you?

I am licensed in Illinois, so if you are in Illinois feel free to call our office at (224) 723-5408. Or check out our website at www.re-medispa.com. Have a wonderful day!

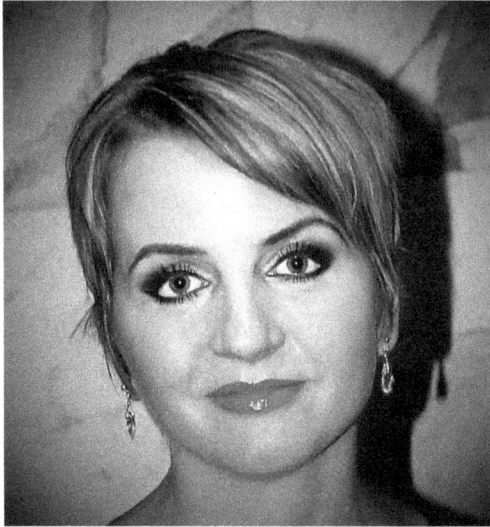

Renata Ciszek APN-BC

info@re-medispa.com

(224) 723-5408

re-medispa.com

666 Dundee Rd #804, Northbrook, IL 60062

www.ingramcontent.com/pod-product-compliance
Lightning Source LLC
Chambersburg PA
CBHW060707280326
41933CB00012B/2343